Anti-Aging

How to Look and Feel Younger

By Kimmy Darlene Nelson

Remain young forever

~ Kimmy Darlene

Nelson Publishing Solutions
392 East Stevens Rd. G13
Palm Springs, CA. 92262

About the Author

Kimmy Nelson has five years of University level education in Health Sciences and over ten years in homeopathy studies and anti-aging research. This book gives simple solutions that can usually be found right in your kitchen cupboards.

She shares information about common illnesses and how to treat them from a holistic approach. She doesn't just tell you ways that you can just treat the symptoms rather gets to the root and tries to remedy it from the starting point.

Rest is essential for the healing properties to manifest speedily. And a healthy environment is also important to get optimal results. Kimmy Nelson guides you to a natural path for anti-aging and health. Using a Healing Approach to master Disease Control and operate in Preventive Health care as well as Traditional and Conventional Medicine applied conservatively.

She shares information on how and when to use a formula from skin care doctors on the best way to remove wrinkles naturally. She also shares information on how to maintain younger looking skin without spending a fortune.

And how to get rid of dark circles under the eyes. She teaches you what causes wrinkles and how to prevent them in a healthy manner. Most of the ingredients can be made from ingredients already in your cupboards or medicine cabinet.

Dedicated to my four beautiful
and ageless sisters~

Wrinkles Are Nothing but Accumulated Dead Skin Cells

In the early nineties was the first time that I ever thought about doing something about a wrinkle. I had heard about alpha hydroxyl and that the juice from fruits could be used as alpha hydroxy in it's natural state.

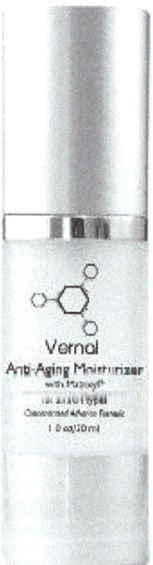

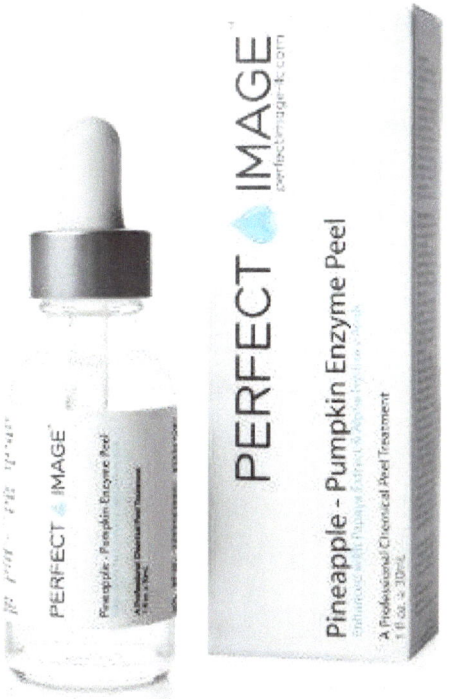

So I put a little fruit juice on a wrinkle and I rubbed it in a circular motion after my professor from "Anatomy & Physiology" had taught us that wrinkles were nothing more than the formation of dead cells.

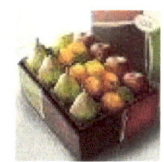

Almost the exact same cellular structure of dead cells that form our hair or finger nails. And that if you could get the old dead cells off of your face then the wrinkle would also vanish or greatly diminish. I tried it and it worked. It worked so well that I have used it ever since.

Only twenty years later my dermatologist found a spot on my shoulder and he removed it.

 Then he told me that I needed to stay out of the sun as much as possible or to use sunscreen all of the time when I am outside.

This "Badger" is an all natural sunscreen with 30 SPF. See a Photo of it on the next page as it would not fit on this page.

A lot of the products we list will be photo shot on the following page as the format will not allowed to go outside of the borders.

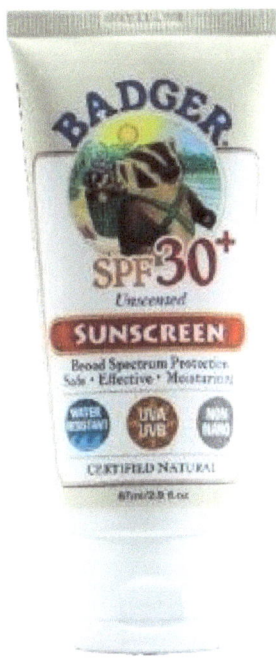

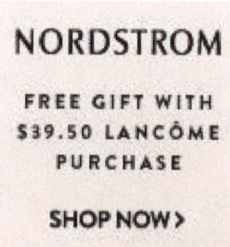
Find more Sunscreen, hats & sunglasses at Nordstrom and take advantage of the "Free Gift" offer too.

In college I took "Fashion & Clothing" too and I learned that there are a couple of things that really cause wrinkles more so then others. The sun causes wrinkles above all else. Secondly, wearing makeup to bed will also age your skin rapidly. Wear Shades!

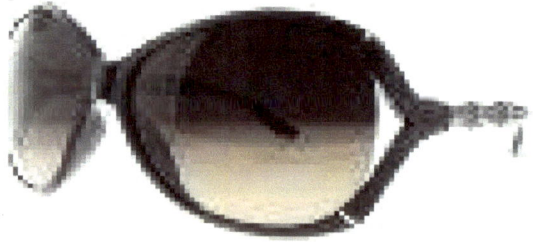

Some people don't like to wear sunscreen or they are simply allergic to it like me. I cannot drive if I put it on because my eyes water so much. So I recommend big sunglasses and a big hat for people who don't want to use sunscreen.

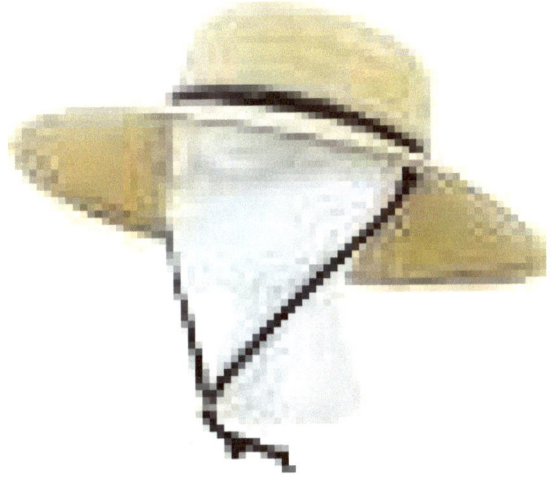

Thirdly, you want to stay away from products that contain mineral oil. I don't think it is wrong to use it on your baby's skin because that is what baby oil is. But I do not recommend it at all for anyone's hands for face if you want the skin to remain wrinkle free.

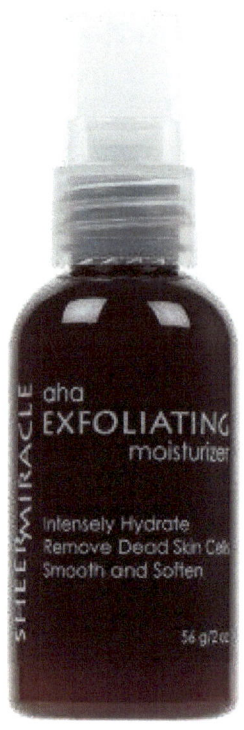

It was not too long after that when I turned on Trinity Broadcast Network and they had a Christian Dermatologist on some program and they were talking about skin protection. He went on to talk about how to get rid of wrinkles by using alpha hydroxy and that it was important to use to use sunscreen.

This one is my Favorite!

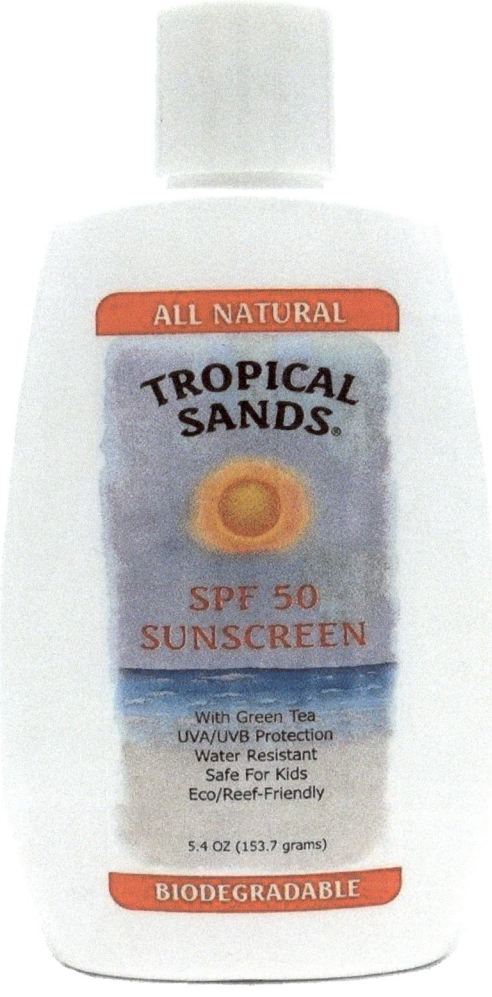

100% All Natural UVA/UVB Protection, Water Resistant, Safe For Kids, Eco/Reef Friendly, SPF 50! This is it!

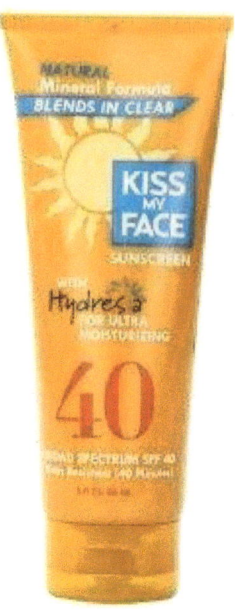

Here is another fine Sun Screen for the face.

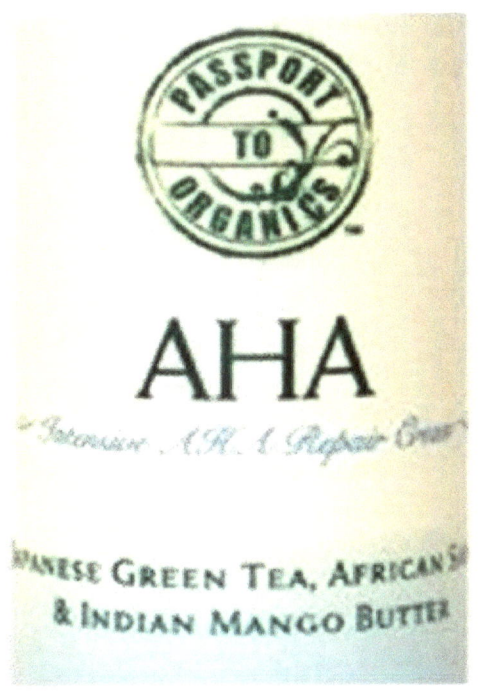

Anytime you use <u>alpha hydroxy</u> you must use sun screen to prevent further damage because now the skin will even be more

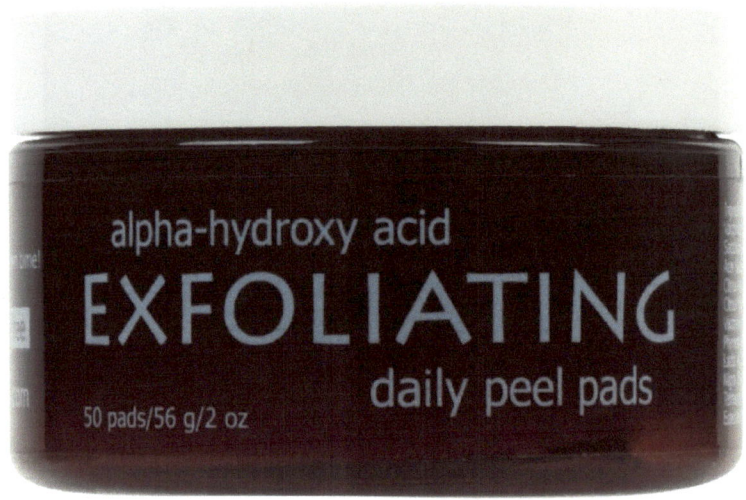

susceptible to the sun as the alpha hydroxy removes some of the top layer of skin.

He said that the best time to use the alpha hydroxy is at night time while we sleep. He said that was when it would be the most effective and the best time to use it if you were going to use it to fight wrinkles.

He also went on to tell us how important it is to use a moisturizer on your skin. He gave a simple recipe that I've been using every since. It is nothing more then

 simple safflower oil or coconut oil combined with raw sugar.

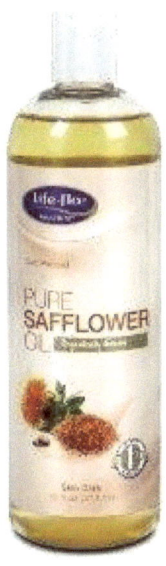

But I am not the kind of person who is going to go to sleep with [raw sugar](#) or sweet on my face because I don't want to attract bugs near my head when I am sleeping. And I found that the sugar and oil mixture is very sticky and the granules of sugar tend to fall off once they are dry and that only makes for a mess.

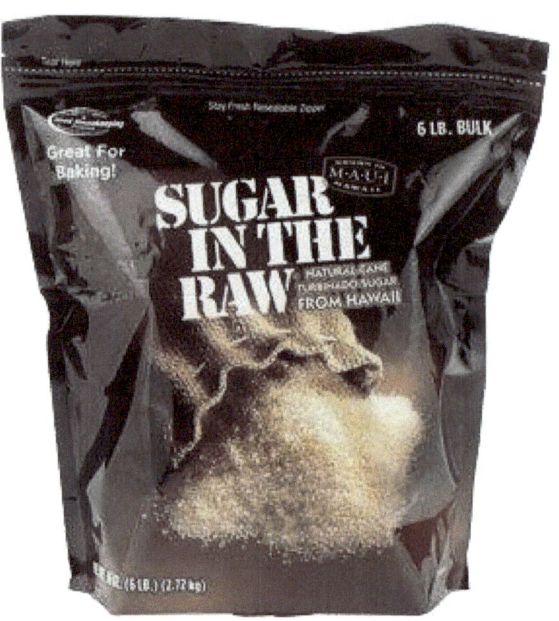

They make alpha hydroxy that you can buy and pay a lot of money for it. But I found that sugar and safflower oil work so much better and they certainly are more assessable and affordable.

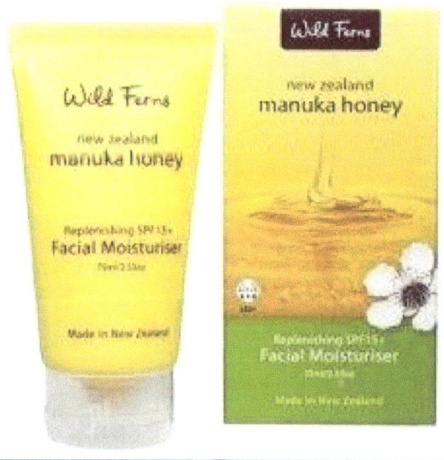

But you can accomplish the same wonderful effects of alpha hydroxy with some natural store bought products like moisturizers with honey in them. Or you could actually just use honey and safflower oil instead of sugar and safflower oil. At least that way it will not turn grainy and fall off. But it can still be too sticky.

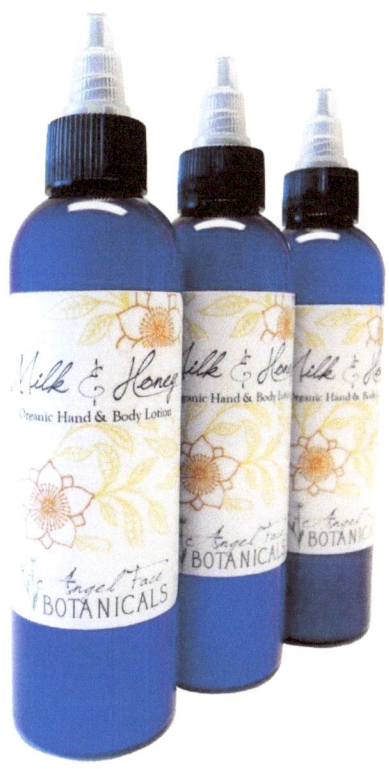

Next you will need to exfoliate on a weekly basis unless the alpha hydroxy that you use has it's own exfoliate in it which a few do.

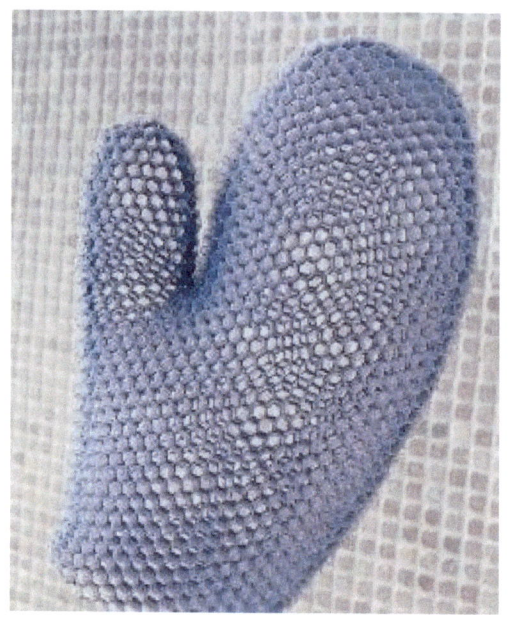

Personally, I use a [hand mit loofa](#) scrub once a week on my face. But you can also just use plain ole corn meal. Or you can try this [Two Speed Rotating Facial Scrub Brush by Olay](#)

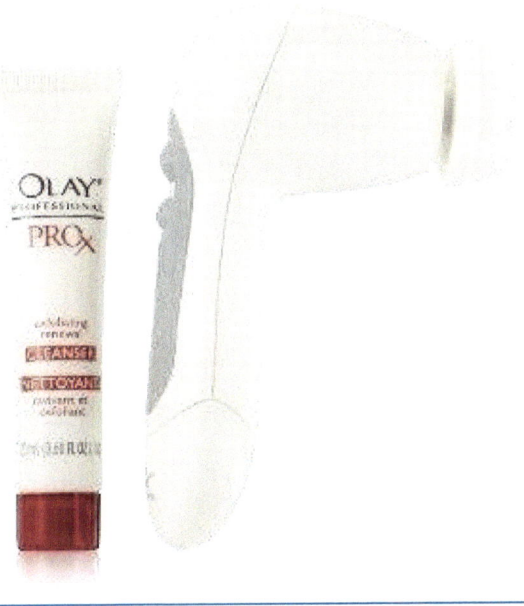

There was a time when I was instructed to just simply use plain ole corn meal and I did. It worked marvelously. And probably had some added benefits besides just removing the dead skin cells. Maybe it had some kind of mineral rejuvinator or anti oxidant effect. I just know it worked.

Red Rooibos always has great all natural skin benefits as it is trace minerals and vitamins in ample supply and it contains a nutrient found in the skin of an egg shell known as "hydroxy acid" or Alpha Hydrox.

Rooibos Tea contains zinc and alpha hydroxy acid which promote healthy skin. And because Rooibos has about fifty times more antioxidants then Green Tea it also reverses the signs of aging from the inside out.

3 Free Samples Beauty Purchase Plus Free Shipping! Online Only at Lord and Taylor! Shop Now!

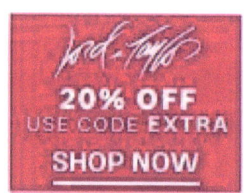

An Employee-Owned Company

moist and light   **easy to prepare**

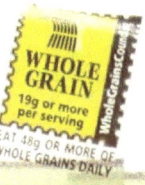

WHEAT FREE
GLUTEN FREE
DAIRY FREE

CORNBREAD MIX

**ALL
NATURAL
PRODUCT**

**YOU CAN
SEE OUR
QUALITY**

BOB'S Red Mill®

Stone ground whole grain cornmeal and sorghum impart an
unmatched flavor and texture from another era to our Gluten Free
Cornbread Mix. After easy preparation you will bake perfectly
moist and light cornbread.

Casein Free   NET WT 20 OZ (1 LB 4 OZ) 567g   K

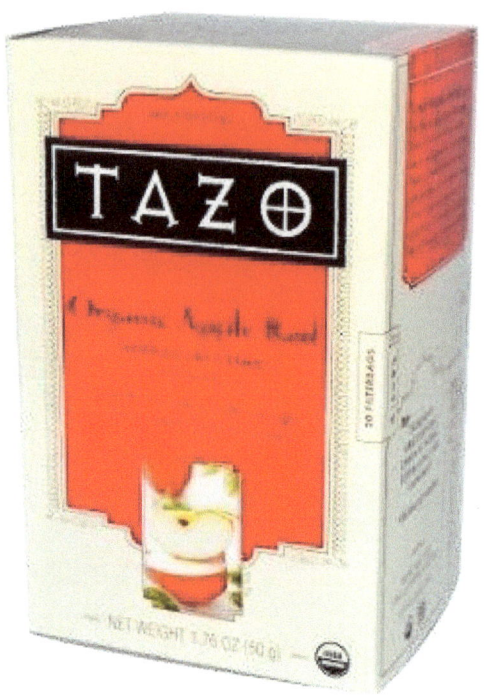

It is also important to have the right lifestyles and food choices that support a healthy skin foundation.

[Vitamin A & D](#) supplements in the oil softgels are great to take orally and to use topically in areas where wrinkles are likely.

That don't smell like roses unless you add a rose scent to cover it but I assure you that it is well worth it. Besides they make other supplements called "[Hope In A Jar](#)"

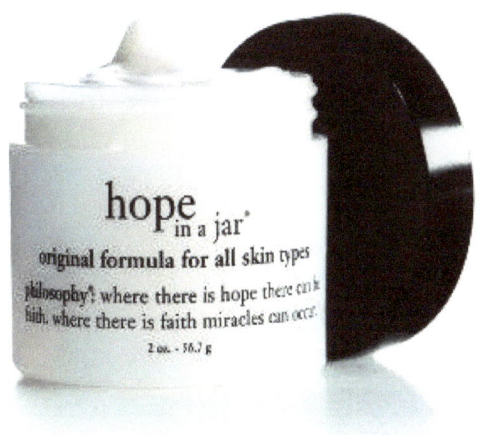

---

or Dianne Younger's facial serum that also have a different smell but the products work!

Here you will see [Orlane Crème Royale Neck and Decollete](#) though I cannot recall the scent of this one. It has remarkable results!

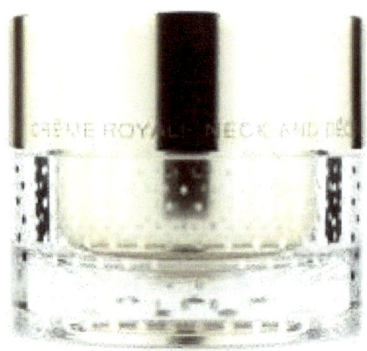

The good thing with Vitamin A & D is that you can put on some scented safflower oil on top of it and it will cover the slight fresh sea scent of the Vitamin A & D.

DMAE is another supplement that has remarkable effects to improve skin appearance. Here you find the DMAE & Arginine Firming Cream. There are some products that acutally contain Rooibos Tea in the topical facial product and application too.

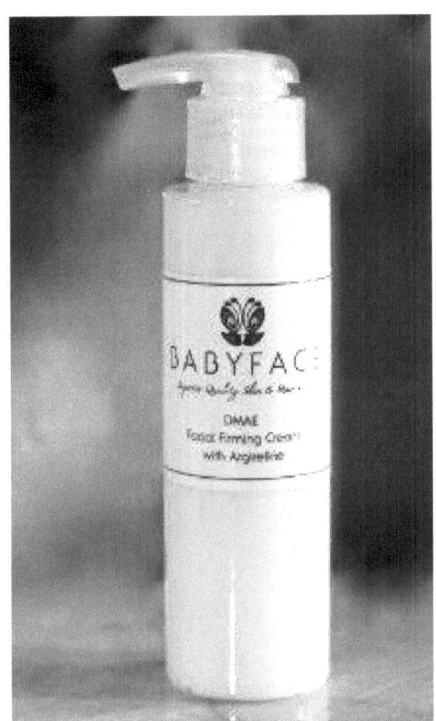

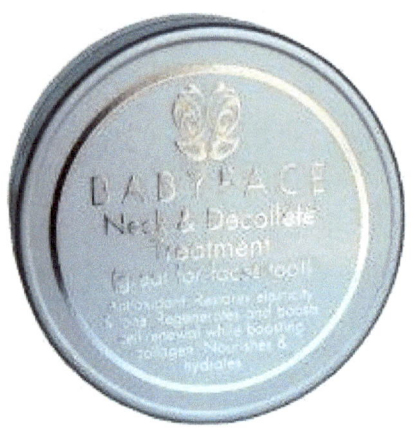

This Is BabyFace Face & Neck Cream with Antioxidants, Peptides, Hydration & Anti-Aging Royal Jelly, Bee Propolis, Argiline, Squaline, Coenzyme Q10, Retinol, Vitamin C

Here is Angel Face Rooibos and MSM Moisturizer

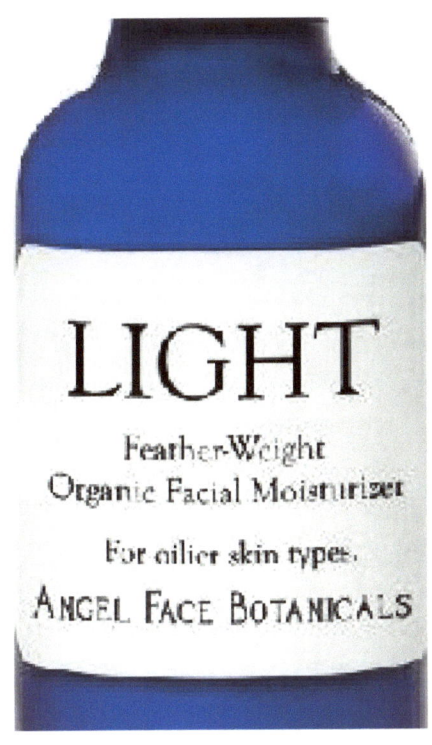

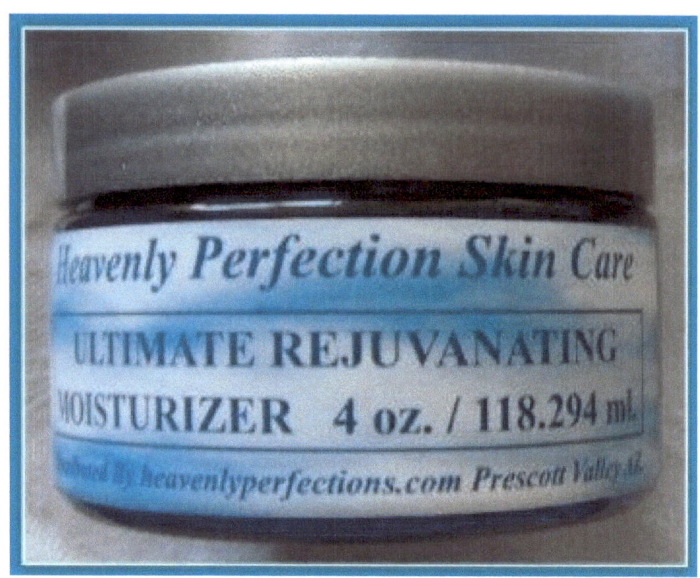

This one is "Heavenly Perfection Skin Care" Ulitmate Rejunanating Moisturizer

It is 81% Organic and contains DMAE, MSM, Rooibos, Pomegranate extracts and Hyaluronic Acid and at a very good price I might add. This is one of the best products that I've listed so far in terms of what you get and cost.

A milk facial is helpful when you need to restore the moisture and supple feel of soft skin. It is always good to have a box of instant milk on hand to bathe with occasionally too.

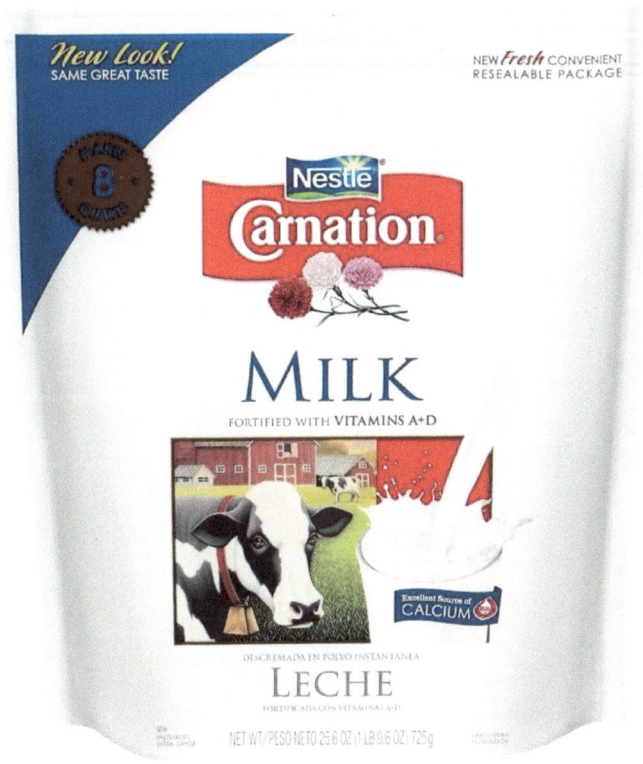

In the bath soak you just add about three cups of powdered milk to a whole large bath tub of water and soak in it for 15 minutes. Rinse off completely in a shower of warm water.

For a facial just apply milk directly to your face using a cotton ball. Leave it for fifteen minutes then rinse with water.

They also make [products with milk](#) in them so you don't have to do all the dirty work.

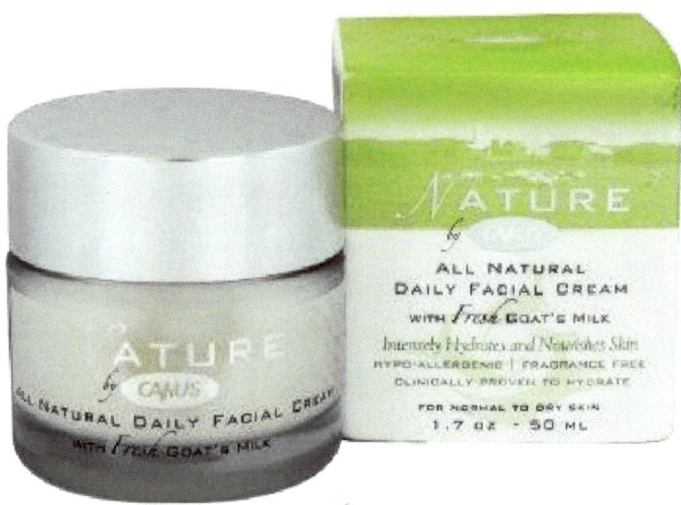

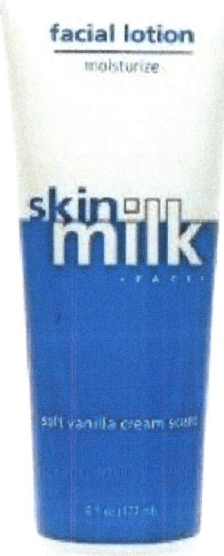

This Skin [Milk has Vanilla Scent](#) to it and makes it especially nice.

Also we have this miracle [scar eraser](#)

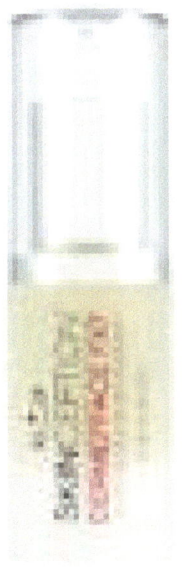

And [Kollagen (Collagen)](Kollagen%20%28Collagen%29)

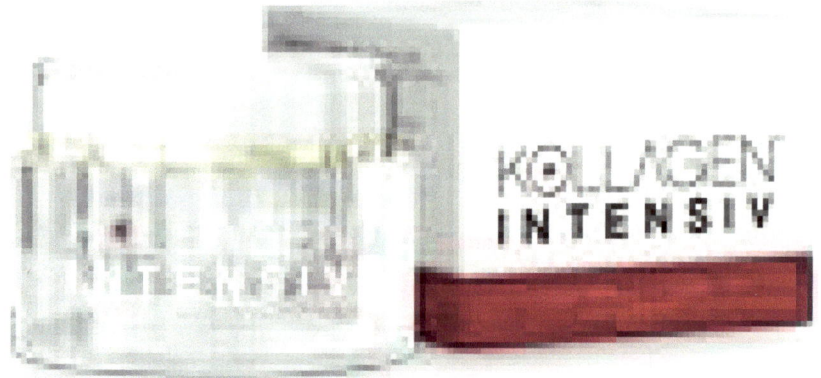

And some have sworn that mineral mud masks like "[Pure](#)" from the Dead Sea brought them renewed youth.

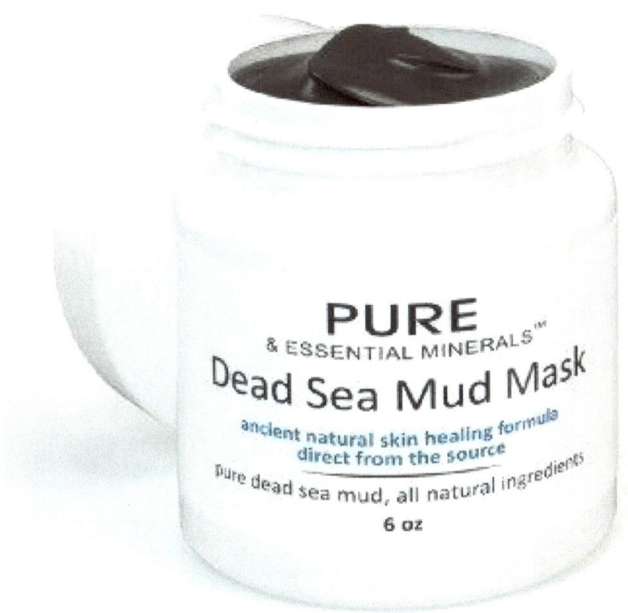

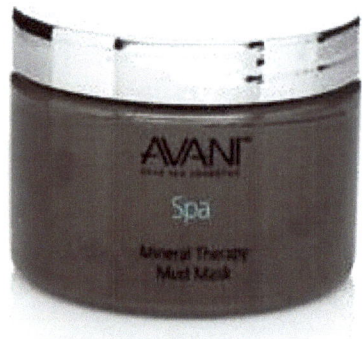

Or In [Avani Mineral Mud Mask](#) from the Dead Sea

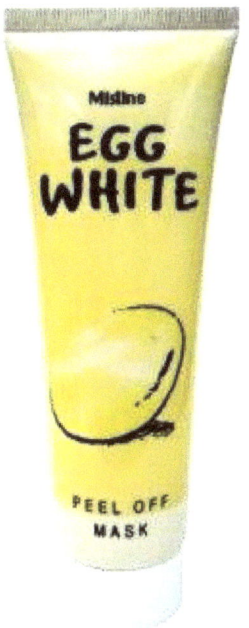

Eggs are particularly good to refine pores and tighten your skin. You can also find them already prepared in some facial products like "Egg White" Peel Off Mask.

Or like the Eggs In [SkinFood Egg White Mask](#) used to refine skin pores and tighten the skin like a face lift.

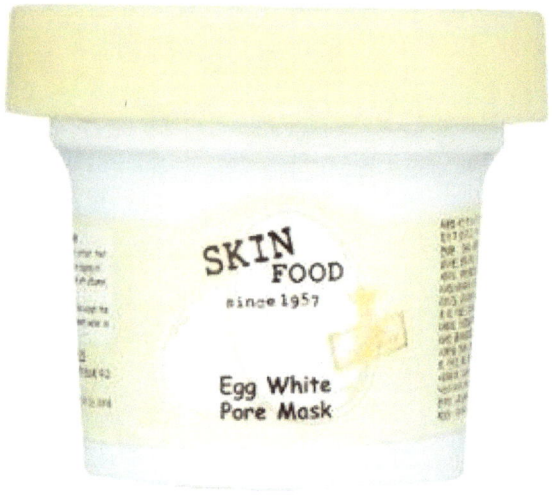

If you have a problem with eyes swelling as I do after I cry or if my nose gets stuffy then you can do as I do. I take [Boswellia](#) and Turmeric or [Bromelain](#) to stop the inflammation from the inside.

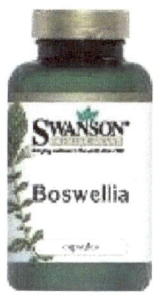

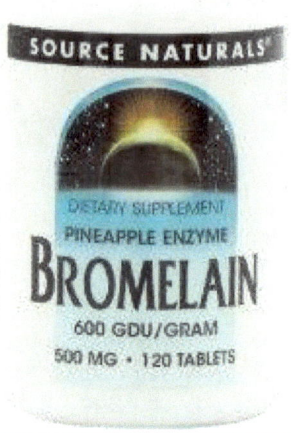

Bromelain stops swelling and inflammation. It is Pineapple Enzyme.

Taken on an empty stomach at the start of each day it can also prevent cancer. You can have water with it but don't eat for another thirty minutes.

Stop eye swelling instantly on the outside by using [Hydrocortisone Cream](#) (NOT OINTMENT)

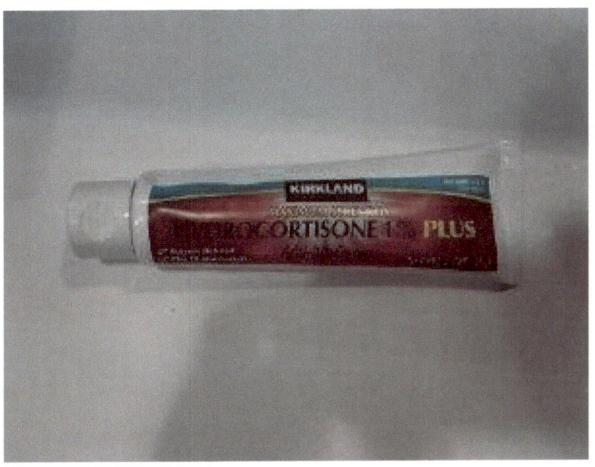

Collagen is really good for the skin. But if you are getting the right amount of Vitamin C every day then your body will produce it's own collagen.

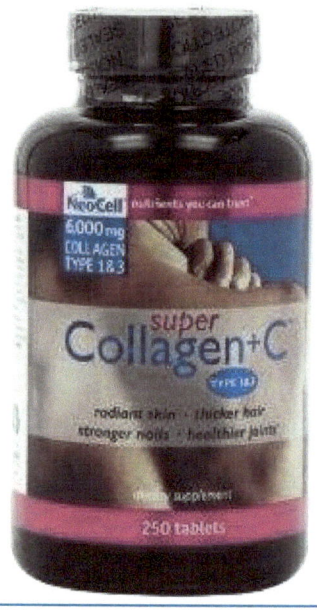

<u>Skinception</u> is another great product for skin lightening on moles, age spots, freckles, birth marks, scars and more!

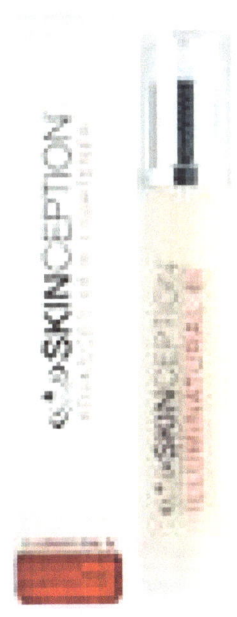

We can thank Dr. Oz for this one! It fills in wrinkles and fine lines from the inside out!

Phyto350

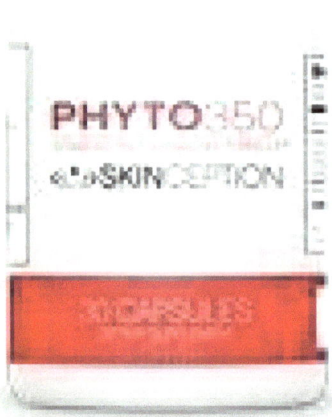

Here is some homeopathic scent of [Lavender](#) that you can add a drop or two to some safflower oil to use on top of the Vitamin A & D softgels once they are applied to the skin.

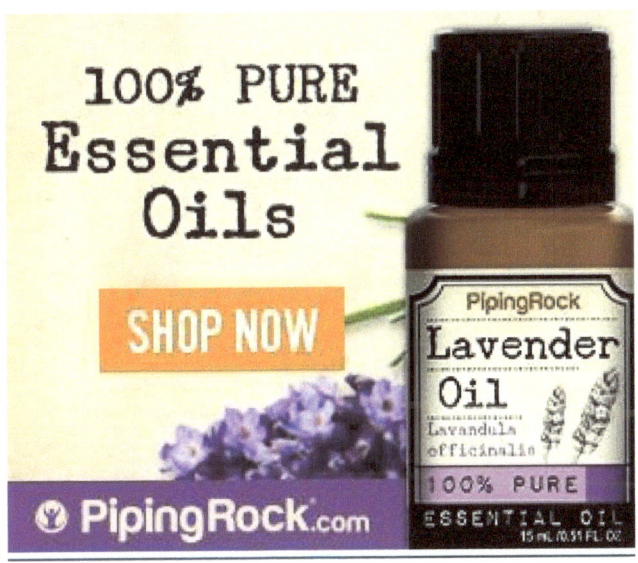

What I Can Do To Effect My Own Aging Process?

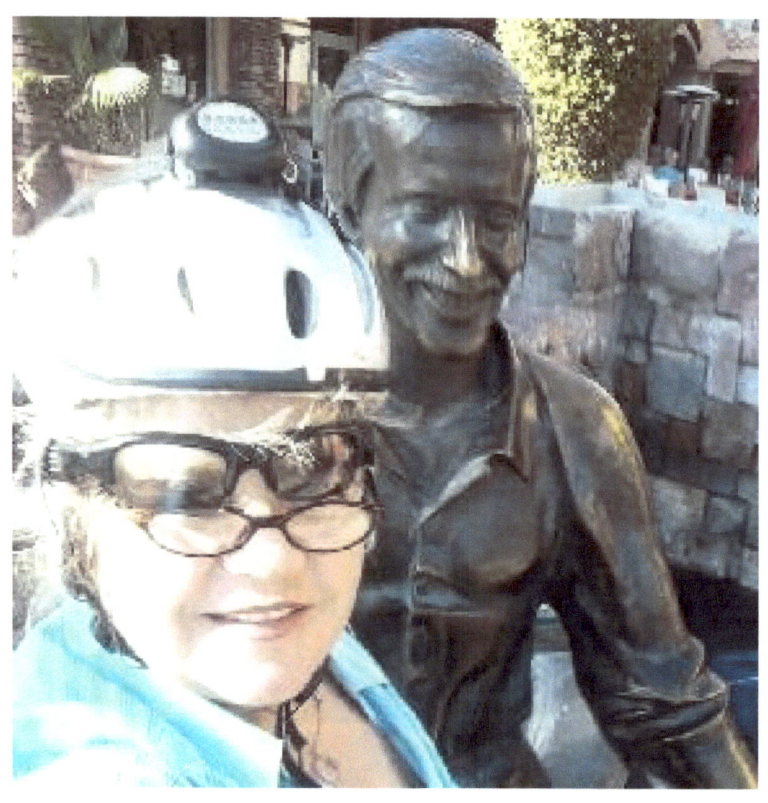

I began eating more healthy foods, removing the not so healthy foods out of my grocery list. I found that if I don't buy them then I cannot use them to cook with or to eat them.

I am hoping that my changed diet will help me progress towards a healthy body day by day, week by week, month by month and year by year. Sometimes it takes time to undo the bad that has been done.

And sometimes it takes time for the new ways to show the benefits of the change. I need to exercise but the pain of the arthritis is so debilitating that I have to take pain medicines and anti-inflammatory medicine just to be able to ride my bike which is the only land exercise that my physical therapists have approved for me.

Now that I know that the sedentary lifestyle is the one that causes disability to worsen, and sedentary lifestyle also prohibits people from recovering from injuries or illness, and sedentary lifestyle also shortens life spans I will fight the pain harder to keep myself active 4 times per week from now on beginning now.

If I ride my bike or do laps in the pool then that will be enough to interrupt the sedentary lifestyle that I have lived for much of the past decade.

I am already over the age of fifty and I've worked very hard on my health by quitting smoking.

I don't live a risky lifestyle of sexual impurity or alcohol consumption.

So the only thing I need to do is to add exercise and continue the other healthy choices that I have made then I can see myself at age seventy in better health than I was at age fifty.

Helpful tips and useful information

"Epidemiologists report that the greatest impact on chronic illness can be made through lifestyle changes rather than technological interventions such as drugs or surgery." (Ferrini & Ferrini

pg.391)

A sedentary lifestyle is associated with many debilitating and life threatening diseases including heart disease, hypertension, obesity, osteoporosis, diabetes, and mental disorders.

It has also been associated with shorter life spans and reduced ability to recover from injuries or illness.

Exercise is used in prevention, treatment and control of high blood pressure. Exercise is also associated with lower risk of early death.

Physical Fitness and Fall Prevention

Balance, endurance, strengthening and flexibility are all important for good health.

Balance exercises can be done by placing your hand on a wall or a chair and doing side and back leg lifts. Also by standing on one foot and by walking heel to toe.

Ten to Fifteen (10-15) repetitions of leg lifts then slowly increase the challenge by removing the chair or the wall to balance.

Endurance can be done by swimming, walking, gardening, raking, or cycling 30 minutes per day five days a week.

Strengthening can be done by free weights or squeeze balls and can prevent falling and maintain functioning through life. Lift a can of soup or a free weight and squeeze a ball two (2) or more days a week for thirty (30) minutes each time.

Start light with elastic bands and you can do 8-12 repetitions for (3) seconds lift or push and hold for one (1) second then release or return for (3) seconds.

Flexibility can be done by stretching all muscle groups before any exercise. Stretch 3-5 times each session hold for 10-30 second while doing it slow and smooth stretches, breath deep and stretch farther each time.

Doing these exercises will help you to maintain physical activity. Think of the ole saying "use it or lose it" to describe the importance of exercise.

We hope that you find lots of healthy and natural ways to remain beautiful inside and out. Thank you!

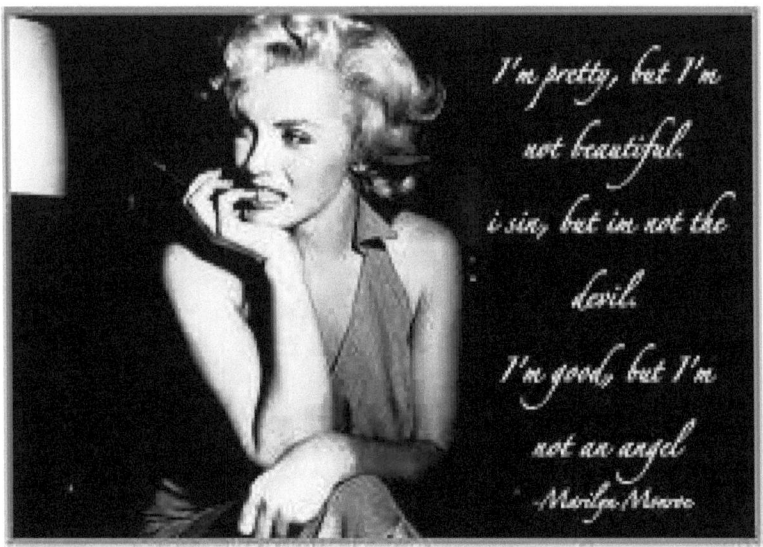

www.ingramcontent.com/pod-product-compliance
Lightning Source LLC
Chambersburg PA
CBHW050826290526
45792CB00001B/274